# MASTERING LIVER CIRRHOSIS

A Comprehensive Guide to Nursing Care Plans
and Management

**Dr. Roy B. Vicknair**

**Copyright © 2024 by Dr. Roy B. Vicknair.**

All rights reserved. No part of this publication may be reproduced, distributed, or transmitted in any form or by any means, including photocopying, recording, or other electronic or mechanical methods, without the prior written permission of the publisher, except in the case of brief quotations embodied in critical reviews and certain other noncommercial uses permitted by copyright law.

# Preface

Liver cirrhosis presents a complex and multifaceted challenge within the realm of healthcare. As a progressive disease, it demands a nuanced and comprehensive approach to patient care. "Mastering Liver Cirrhosis: A Comprehensive Guide to Nursing Care Plans and Management" aims to equip healthcare professionals with the knowledge and tools necessary to deliver exceptional care to patients battling this condition.

This guide delves into the intricacies of liver cirrhosis, offering detailed insights into nursing assessments, interventions, goals, and diagnoses. Each section is meticulously tailored to address the unique needs of patients suffering from liver cirrhosis, ensuring that nursing professionals can provide specialized and effective care.

Within these pages, you will find evidence-based strategies designed to enhance patient outcomes and improve quality of life. From initial assessments to the implementation of comprehensive care plans, this resource serves as a vital tool in the hands of those dedicated to the field of nursing.

By integrating the latest research and clinical practices, "Mastering Liver Cirrhosis" stands as a testament to the importance of specialized nursing care. It is our hope that this guide will not only inform but also inspire healthcare professionals to continually strive for excellence in their practice.

**Dr. Roy B. Vicknair**

Contents

1. What is Liver Cirrhosis?
2. Nursing Care Plans and Management
3. Nursing Problem Priorities
4. Nursing Assessment
5. Nursing Diagnosis
6. Nursing Goals
7. Nursing Interventions and Actions
   -Enhancing Nutritional Balance
   -Managing Ascites and Fluid Volume
   -Providing Skin Care and Promoting Skin Integrity
   -Improving Breathing Pattern and Preventing Respiratory Complications
   -Promoting Safety and Preventing Injury
   -Preventing Hepatic Encephalopathy
   -Promoting Positive Self-Body Image

-Initiating Patient Education and Health Teachings

-Administering Medications and Providing Pharmacologic Support

.-Monitoring Results of Diagnostic and Laboratory Procedures

Abbreviations

1. ADLs - Activities of Daily Living
2. ALT - Alanine Aminotransferase
3. AST- Aspartate Aminotransferase
4. BP - Blood Pressure
5. CBC - Complete Blood Count
6. CIWA - Clinical Institute Withdrawal Assessment
7. CNS- Central Nervous System
8. CT - Computed Tomography

9. DM - Diabetes Mellitus

10. ECG - Electrocardiogram

11. EGD - Esophagogastroduodenoscopy

12. GI - Gastrointestinal

13. HCC - Hepatocellular Carcinoma

14. HE - Hepatic Encephalopathy

15. Hgb - Hemoglobin

16. HR - Heart Rate

17. INR - International Normalized Ratio

18. IV - Intravenous

19. LFTs - Liver Function Tests

20. MELD - Model for End-Stage Liver Disease

21. MRI - Magnetic Resonance Imaging

22. Na+ - Sodium

23. NPO - Nil Per Os (nothing by mouth)

24. NSAIDs - Nonsteroidal Anti-Inflammatory Drugs

25. PE - Physical Examination

26. PT - Prothrombin Time

27. PTT - Partial Thromboplastin Time

28. RN - Registered Nurse

29. RR - Respiratory Rate

30. SBP - Spontaneous Bacterial Peritonitis

31. SGPT - Serum Glutamic-Pyruvic Transaminase

32. SPO2 - Saturation of Peripheral Oxygen

33. TIPS - Transjugular Intrahepatic Portosystemic Shunt

34. TPN - Total Parenteral Nutrition

35. US - Ultrasound

## What is Liver Cirrhosis?

Liver cirrhosis, or hepatic cirrhosis, is a chronic liver disease characterized by widespread destruction and fibrotic regeneration of liver cells. The liver can be damaged by various factors, including viral infections, toxins, hereditary conditions, or autoimmune processes. With each injury, scar tissue (fibrosis) forms, initially without functional loss. Over time, extensive fibrosis replaces most of the liver tissue, leading to cirrhosis and loss of liver function (Farci, 2022). This progressive disease disrupts the liver's structure and vasculature, impairs blood and lymph flow, and ultimately results in hepatic insufficiency.

## Clinical Types of Cirrhosis

Laennec's Cirrhosis: This is the most prevalent form, affecting 30% to 50% of cirrhosis patients. A significant proportion (up to 90%) have a history of chronic alcoholism. Liver damage is primarily due to malnutrition, particularly protein deficiency, combined with prolonged alcohol consumption. Fibrosis develops in the portal areas and around the central veins.

Biliary Cirrhosis: Accounting for 15% to 20% of cases, this type is caused by liver injury or long-term obstruction of the bile ducts.

Postnecrotic Cirrhosis: This type results from various forms of hepatitis, leading to extensive liver cell death and subsequent fibrosis.

Pigment Cirrhosis: Arising from disorders such as hemochromatosis, this form involves the accumulation of excessive iron in the liver.

Idiopathic Cirrhosis: This type has no identifiable cause.

Noncirrhotic Fibrosis: This condition can be due to schistosomiasis, congenital hepatic fibrosis, or idiopathic origins.

## Clinical Presentation and Management of Cirrhosis

**Clinical Presentation:**

Some patients with cirrhosis may be asymptomatic and enjoy a relatively normal life expectancy, while others experience severe symptoms associated with end-stage liver disease, significantly impacting their survival prospects. Common signs and symptoms include:

- Hepatomegaly
- Abdominal pain
- Ascites
- Abdominal distention
- Bulging flanks
- Shifting dullness

- Anorexia

- Weight loss

- Fatigue

- Muscle wasting

Cutaneous Manifestations:

- Jaundice

- Spider angiomata

- Skin telangiectasia (often described as "paper money skin")

- Palmar erythema

- White nails

- Disappearance of lunulae

- Finger clubbing (Wolf & Anand, 2020)

## Nursing Care Plans and Management

The primary goals of nursing care for patients with liver cirrhosis are to manage symptoms such as ascites, jaundice, and encephalopathy, reduce the risk of injury, prevent and treat complications like portal hypertension and variceal bleeding, and promote self-care and education to enhance overall health outcomes. Nursing interventions include:

- Monitoring and promoting adequate nutrition and fluid balance
- Addressing the psychological and emotional needs of patients and their families

### Nursing Problem Priorities

Key nursing priorities for patients with liver cirrhosis include:

1. Managing and Monitoring Liver Function: Regularly assess liver function to detect and address deterioration.
2. Addressing Complications: Focus on complications like portal hypertension and ascites.
3. Providing Supportive Care: Alleviate symptoms and improve the patient's quality of life.
4. Patient Education: Instruct patients on dietary changes and fluid restrictions as needed.
5. Administering Medications: Manage symptoms and slow disease progression through appropriate pharmacologic interventions.

6. Managing Complications: Monitor for and treat conditions such as hepatic encephalopathy and variceal bleeding.

7. Counseling and Support: Encourage lifestyle modifications, including alcohol cessation and weight management.

## Nursing Assessment

Subjective and Objective Data to Assess:

- Complaints of fatigue and weakness
- Reports of abdominal pain or discomfort
- Presence of ascites, indicated by abdominal distension and shifting dullness on percussion
- Nausea, vomiting, or changes in appetite

- A history of alcohol misuse or binge drinking
- Reports of jaundice (yellowing of the skin and eyes)
- Presence of pruritus (itching)
- Reports of weight loss or changes in body weight
- History of coagulation disorders or easy bruising

- Signs of hepatic encephalopathy, such as altered mental status, confusion, or asterixis (flapping tremor)
- Presence of spider angiomas (dilated blood vessels) or palmar erythema (reddening of the palms)
- Elevated liver enzymes (ALT, AST), bilirubin, and INR (international normalized ratio)

## Nursing Diagnosis

After conducting a comprehensive assessment, the nurse formulates a diagnosis to address the specific challenges posed by liver cirrhosis. This diagnosis is based on clinical judgment and a thorough understanding of the patient's health condition. Although nursing diagnoses provide a framework for organizing care, their applicability may vary in different clinical situations. In practice, the use of specific diagnostic labels may not be as prominent as other components of the care plan. The nurse's clinical expertise and judgment are crucial in developing a care plan tailored to the unique needs and priorities of each patient.

## Nursing Goals

Goals and expected outcomes for patients with liver cirrhosis may include:

- The patient will demonstrate progressive weight gain, with lab values normalizing appropriately.
- The patient will show no further signs of malnutrition.
- The patient will maintain stabilized fluid volume, with balanced intake and output, stable weight, normal vital signs, and no edema.
- The patient will preserve skin integrity.
- The patient will report reduced itching or the ability to tolerate itching without scratching.
- The patient will identify personal risk factors and employ techniques to prevent skin breakdown.

- The patient will maintain an effective respiratory pattern, be free of dyspnea and cyanosis, with arterial blood gasses (ABGs) and vital capacity within acceptable ranges.
- The patient will maintain homeostasis, with no bleeding incidents.
- The patient will adopt behaviors to reduce the risk of bleeding.
- The patient will sustain normal mentation and orientation.
- The patient will implement lifestyle changes to prevent or minimize the recurrence of problems.
- The patient will verbalize understanding and acceptance of self in their current situation.
- The patient will express feelings and methods for coping with negative self-perception.
- The patient will demonstrate understanding of the disease process, prognosis, and potential complications.

- The patient will identify and initiate necessary lifestyle changes and actively participate in their care.

## Nursing Interventions and Actions

Therapeutic Interventions and Nursing Actions for Liver Cirrhosis Patients:

1. Enhancing Nutritional Balance

   - Early recognition and treatment of malnutrition are crucial in managing patients with liver disease, from compensated cirrhosis to liver failure. With the increasing prevalence of obesity, diabetes, and their link to non-alcoholic fatty liver disease (NAFLD), nutritional imbalances are more frequently observed in cirrhosis patients. The coexistence of adiposity and sarcopenia, known as sarcopenic obesity, presents unique nutritional challenges in optimizing metabolic risk factors and muscle function (Dhaliwal et al., 2020).

## Evaluation and Assessment of Malnutrition in Liver Cirrhosis Patients

**Evaluate for Malnutrition:**

A significant portion (80-90%) of the blood exiting the stomach and intestines carries nutrients to the liver for conversion into usable substances. Patients with liver dysfunction frequently suffer from malnutrition due to poor dietary choices, a preference for alcohol over food, or malabsorption syndromes. Factors contributing to malnutrition include the liver's inability to process or digest nutrients, anorexia, nausea, vomiting, indigestion, and early satiety due to ascites. Additionally, reduced bile secretion can impair the absorption of fats and fat-soluble vitamins (A, D, E, and K).

Assess Interest in Eating and Ability to Chew, Swallow, and Taste:
Evaluate factors affecting nutrient ingestion and digestion. Patients with significant ascites may have abdominal discomfort, reduced appetite, and decreased oral intake. Anorexia is common and may be exacerbated by the direct pressure of ascites on the gastrointestinal tract (Wolf & Anand, 2020).

Utilize Nutritional Screening Tools:
All patients with liver cirrhosis, regardless of BMI, should be screened for malnutrition using validated tools such as the Malnutrition Universal Screening Tool (MUST) and the Nutritional Risk Screening-2002 (NRS-2002) (Dhaliwal et al., 2020).

Assess Functional Status:

Evaluate the patient's functional status upon consultation. Observe whether they walk unaided, their handshake strength, and their ability to rise from a chair. Assess performance in daily activities and perceived exercise tolerance. Specific measures of functional ability in cirrhosis include the short physical performance battery, incremental shuttle walk tests, and the liver frailty index, which includes hand grip strength, timed chair stands, and balance (Dhaliwal et al., 2020).

Measure Dietary Intake by Calorie Count:

Track dietary intake to understand needs and deficiencies. Patients with cirrhosis require a balanced protein diet, providing 2,000 to 3,000 calories daily for liver cell regeneration. For compensated cirrhosis, the recommended energy intake is 25-35 kcal/kg/day, with a protein intake of 1.2-1.5 g/kg/day to maintain muscle mass. For decompensated cirrhosis with sarcopenia, the energy intake recommendation is 30-35 kcal/kg/day, and protein intake is 1.5-2.0 g/kg/day to prevent further muscle loss and reverse sarcopenia (Dhaliwal et al., 2020).

Weigh the Patient as Indicated:
Regularly monitor weight, fluid status, recent weight history, and skinfold measurements. Weight alone may not accurately reflect nutritional status due to the presence of edema and/or ascites. Skinfold measurements can help assess changes in muscle mass and subcutaneous fat reserves. Record dry body weight and BMI, using post-paracentesis weight or estimating by subtracting percentages based on the severity of

ascites (mild: 5%; moderate: 10%; severe: 15%) and peripheral edema (5% if bilateral) (Dhaliwal et al., 2020).

Performing Anthropometric Measurements:
Conduct anthropometric assessments to measure muscle mass (Mid-Arm Muscle Circumference [MAMC]) and contractile function (hand grip strength), both predictors of mortality. Measure hand grip strength three times in the non-dominant hand and compare with standard values for women (29 kg) and men (40 kg). Obtain MAMC by measuring the mid-arm circumference (MAC), which includes muscle and adipose tissue, and triceps skinfold, which estimates adipose thickness (Dhaliwal et al., 2020).

Assess the Severity of Cirrhosis:

Evaluate cirrhosis severity using established prognostic tools. The Child-Turcotte-Pugh (CTP) system has historically been used to predict life expectancy in advanced cirrhosis. A CTP score of 10 or higher correlates with a 50% mortality rate within one year. Since 2002, U.S. liver transplant programs have employed the Model for End-stage Liver Disease (MELD) scoring system to determine the severity of liver disease (Wolf & Anand, 2020).

Monitor Laboratory Studies:
Regularly check serum glucose, prealbumin, albumin, total protein, prothrombin time (PT), and ammonia levels. Refer to Laboratory and Diagnostic Procedures for detailed guidelines.

Review Glycemic Control:

Examine the patient's glycemic control, especially if diabetes and anti-diabetic medications are involved. Utilize Hemoglobin A1c (HbA1c) as a direct marker of glycemic control, but interpret with caution in the presence of anemia, as it may give misleadingly reassuring results (Dhaliwal et al., 2020).

Evaluate the Client for Malnutrition:
Monitor weight changes, fluid status, recent weight history, and skinfold measurements. Weight alone may not accurately reflect nutritional status due to edema and ascites. Skinfold measurements are useful for assessing changes in muscle mass and subcutaneous fat reserves. Record dry body weight and BMI, using post-paracentesis weight or estimating by subtracting percentages based on the severity of

ascites (mild: 5%; moderate: 10%; severe: 15%) and peripheral edema (5% if bilateral) (Dhaliwal et al., 2020).

Perform Anthropometric Measurements:

Assess muscle mass (Mid-Arm Muscle Circumference [MAMC]) and contractile function (hand grip strength), both of which predict mortality. Measure hand grip strength three times in the non-dominant hand and compare with standard values for women (29 kg) and men (40 kg). Obtain MAMC by measuring the mid-arm circumference (MAC), which includes muscle and adipose tissue, and triceps skinfold, which estimates adipose thickness (Dhaliwal et al., 2020).

Assess the Severity of Cirrhosis:

Evaluate cirrhosis severity using established prognostic tools. The Child-Turcotte-Pugh (CTP) system has historically been used to predict life expectancy in advanced cirrhosis. A CTP score of 10 or higher correlates with a 50% mortality rate within one year. Since 2002, U.S. liver transplant programs have employed the Model for End-stage Liver Disease (MELD) scoring system to determine the severity of liver disease (Wolf & Anand, 2020).

Monitor Laboratory Studies:
Regularly check serum glucose, prealbumin, albumin, total protein, prothrombin time (PT), and ammonia levels. Refer to Laboratory and Diagnostic Procedures for detailed guidelines.

Review Glycemic Control:

Examine the patient's glycemic control, especially if diabetes and anti-diabetic medications are involved. Utilize Hemoglobin A1c (HbA1c) as a direct marker of glycemic control, but interpret with caution in the presence of anemia, as it may give misleadingly reassuring results (Dhaliwal et al., 2020).

Encourage Eating and Explain Dietary Reasons: Motivate the patient to eat and explain the rationale behind specific dietary choices. Assist the patient during meals if they tire easily, or enlist the help of a family caregiver. Involve the patient in meal planning to accommodate their food preferences. Improved nutrition is crucial for recovery. The patient may eat better with family involvement and preferred foods. Encourage a regular eating pattern of meals and snacks every 2 to 3 hours, including a bedtime snack, to reduce starvation periods and minimize muscle and fat breakdown for metabolic fuel (Dhaliwal et al., 2020).

**Encourage Consuming All Meals and Supplements:**

Patients may eat minimally due to disinterest, nausea, weakness, or malaise. The 2010 practice guidelines for alcoholic liver disease by the American Association for the Study of Liver Disease and the American College of Gastroenterology recommend aggressive treatment of protein-calorie malnutrition in alcoholic cirrhosis patients. They suggest multiple daily feedings, including breakfast and a nighttime snack (Wolf & Anand, 2020).

**Provide Small, Frequent Meals:**

Due to increased intra-abdominal pressure and ascites, patients may poorly tolerate larger meals. For energy malnutrition, recommend divided meals and late evening snacks, such as rice balls, liquid nutrients, and branch chain amino acids (BCAA) enriched supplements. Approximately 200 kcal should be taken as a snack before bedtime to reduce nighttime starvation. These snacks should be easy to prepare and consume (Dhaliwal et al., 2020).

Offer Salt Substitutes, if Permitted:
Salt substitutes can enhance food flavor and increase appetite; however, avoid those containing ammonium to reduce the risk of encephalopathy. Initial therapy often involves salt restriction, with diets containing less than 2000 mg of sodium daily. Some patients with refractory ascites may need a diet with less than

500 mg of sodium daily. Ensure patients do not create diets that risk calorie-protein malnutrition (Wolf & Anand, 2020).

Restrict Alcohol, Raw/Uncooked Foods, and Excessively Fatty Foods:
Alcohol is unsafe for patients with cirrhosis as it can further damage the liver and contribute to malnutrition. Patients with alcohol dependence may prioritize drinking over eating nutritious foods. Liver damage affects bile production, impairing the processing of high-fat meals. Furthermore, individuals with liver cirrhosis have compromised immune systems, leaving them vulnerable to bacteria and viruses found in raw or undercooked food (Daniel, 2022).

Encourage Frequent Mouth Care, Especially Before Meals:

Clients often experience sore or bleeding gums and an unpleasant taste in the mouth, which can lead to decreased appetite. Fetor hepaticus, a condition associated with portal hypertension and portosystemic shunts, causes breath to have a sweet, musty, and sometimes fecal odor (Thomas, 2021).

Promote Undisturbed Rest Periods, Especially Before Meals:
Rest helps conserve energy, reducing metabolic demands on the liver and promoting cellular regeneration. Energy balance, which includes resting energy expenditure, physical activity, and thermogenesis, is crucial. Despite reduced physical activity in cirrhotic patients, their total energy expenditure ranges from 28 to 37.5 kcal/kg body weight per day (Dhaliwal et al., 2020).

Recommend Smoking Cessation and Educate on Its Negative Effects:

Reducing gastric stimulation and irritation decreases the risk of bleeding. Smoking negatively impacts the liver through toxic, immunologic, and oncogenic mechanisms. Therefore, cessation is essential to prevent further liver damage (Rutledge & Asgharpour, 2020).

Maintain NPO Status When Indicated:

Gastrointestinal rest may be necessary for acutely ill patients to decrease liver demands and lower ammonia and urea production. During NPO status, nutrition must be provided enterally or parenterally. To avoid caloric deficits, advance the diet as soon as possible and use an

NG tube for enteral nutrition if necessary (Martin & Stotts, 2020).

Refer to a Dietitian for Nutritional Management: A dietitian can design a high-calorie, low-fat, moderate-to-high protein diet with simple carbohydrates, limiting sodium and fluids as needed. Liquid supplements may be required. High-calorie foods are essential due to typically limited intake. Carbohydrates provide immediate energy, while fats are poorly absorbed and may cause discomfort. Proteins are crucial for improving serum protein levels, reducing edema, and promoting liver cell regeneration. If ammonia levels are elevated or if hepatic encephalopathy is present, restrict proteins and ammonia-rich foods like gelatin. Patients may better tolerate vegetable proteins than meat proteins.

Provide Tube Feedings, TPN, and Lipids if Indicated:

Tube feedings, total parenteral nutrition (TPN), and lipid supplements may be necessary to supplement the diet or provide nutrients when clients are unable to eat due to nausea, anorexia, or interference from esophageal varices. Naso- or orogastric tube placement is typically safe post-intubation for clients without active gastrointestinal bleeding, regardless of variceal history. Parenteral feeding should only be used if enteral feeding cannot meet the client's energy needs or is not feasible (Martin & Stotts, 2020).

Optimize Protein Intake as Recommended:

Optimizing protein intake is crucial due to increased total body protein breakdown and reduced muscle protein synthesis. Clients should aim for at least 3 to 4 servings of high-protein foods daily, such as eggs and lean meats (Dhaliwal et al., 2020).

Provide Nutritional Oral Supplements as Prescribed:
Meeting calorie and protein requirements can be challenging, especially for clients with sarcopenia, necessitating the use of nutritional supplements. These typically include low-volume, high-protein sip feeds tailored to individual needs. A daily multivitamin (excluding manganese, which may exacerbate hepatic encephalopathy in cirrhotic clients) should be considered, with adjustments for specific vitamin and mineral deficiencies in malnourished or decompensated states (Martin & Stotts, 2020).

Encourage Physical Activities as Tolerated:

Encouraging physical activity and exercise is beneficial for managing weight and improving muscle mass and strength. Exercise programs should be tailored to individual capabilities, including warm-ups, a mix of aerobic and resistance exercises, and cool-downs for balance and flexibility training. Moderate-intensity activities are recommended, allowing clients to speak in short sentences during exertion (Dhaliwal et al., 2020).

## Managing Ascites and Fluid Volume

Ascites can be caused by hepatic or nonhepatic diseases and is defined by an accumulation of excess fluid in the peritoneal cavity. Patients with cirrhosis often experience sodium and water retention, impaired excretion of free water, and intravascular volume overload. These abnormalities can occur despite normal glomerular filtration rate and are partly due to elevated levels of renin and aldosterone (Wolf & Anand, 2020).

- Evaluate respiratory status, observing for increased respiratory rate and dyspnea. These symptoms may indicate pulmonary congestion. The following conditions are associated with cirrhosis: lower oxygen saturation, ventilation-perfusion mismatch, hepatic hydrothorax, portopulmonary hypertension, decreased pulmonary diffusion capacity, and hyperventilation (Farci, 2022).

- Auscultate lungs, noting diminished breath sounds and adventitious sounds development. Increasing pulmonary congestion can lead to consolidation, impaired gas exchange, and complications. Most patients with hepatopulmonary syndrome (HPS) present with dyspnea, orthopnea, platypnea, and cyanosis. Platypnea or orthodeoxia refers to worsening breathlessness when sitting or standing, relieved by lying down (Amer & Elsiesy, 2017).

- Monitor blood pressure (and central venous pressure if available). Observe for jugular venous distention and distended abdominal veins. Elevated blood pressure usually indicates fluid volume excess but may not manifest due to fluid shifts out of the vascular space. Distension of external jugular and abdominal veins indicates vascular congestion. Portal hypertension results from increased portal venous inflow and resistance to portal blood flow. Patients with cirrhosis demonstrate increased splanchnic arterial flow and subsequent venous inflow into the liver, influenced by decreased peripheral vascular resistance and increased cardiac output (Wolf & Anand, 2020).

- Monitor for cardiac dysrhythmias. Auscultate heart sounds, noting the presence of S3/S4 gallop rhythm. These may result from heart failure, decreased coronary arterial perfusion, and electrolyte imbalances. Physical examination may reveal accentuated and split-second heart sounds, right ventricular heave, right-sided S3 gallop, jugular vein distention, and lower extremity edema suggestive of portopulmonary hypertension (Benz et al., 2020).

- Assess for signs indicating ascites presence. Approximately 1500 ml of fluid is required for reliable detection of ascites by physical examination; diagnostic accuracy is significantly reduced in obese patients. Signs such as shifting dullness, fluid wave, and puddle signs support the diagnosis, with shifting dullness demonstrating 83% sensitivity and 56% specificity in detecting ascites.

- Evaluate the extent of peripheral edema. Fluid shifts into tissues due to sodium and water retention, decreased albumin levels, and elevated antidiuretic hormone (ADH). Bilateral edema may result from portal vein congestion, increasing capillary permeability, and decreasing plasma oncotic pressure due to reduced albumin synthesis by the liver (Goyal et al., 2022).

Measure Intake and Output (I&O), Perform Daily Weighing, and Monitor Weight Gain Exceeding 0.5 kg/day

These assessments evaluate the client's circulating volume status, fluid shifts development or resolution, and response to treatment. Positive fluid balance or weight gain often indicates ongoing fluid retention. Decreased circulating volume due to fluid shifts can directly impact renal function and urine output, potentially leading to hepatorenal syndrome. Clients with alcohol dependence frequently exhibit fluid retention and ascites. Severe generalized edema can result in significant weight gain for the client (Tanaka et al., 2021).

Assess Abdominal Girth

Measuring abdominal girth reflects fluid accumulation (ascites) resulting from the loss of plasma proteins/fluid into the peritoneal space. Excessive fluid accumulation can decrease circulating volume, indicating signs of dehydration. A correlation between pre-paracentesis girth and ascitic weight has been identified, aiding in ascitic weight estimation and dry weight calculation, particularly when paracentesis isn't feasible or when nutritional assessment requires dry weight (Lamarti & Hickson, 2019).

Monitor Serum Albumin and Electrolytes (Potassium and Sodium)

Reduced serum albumin levels affect plasma colloid osmotic pressure, contributing to edema formation. Changes in renal blood flow, elevated levels of ADH and aldosterone, and diuretic use to reduce total body water can lead to electrolyte imbalances. Ascitic fluid protein and albumin levels are measured alongside serum albumin to calculate the serum-ascites albumin gradient. A gradient equal to or greater than 1.1 g/dL indicates portal hypertension with 97% accuracy (JI, 2022).

## Monitor Sequential Chest X-rays and Other Imaging Studies

Clients frequently experience vascular congestion, pulmonary edema, and pleural effusions. Chest X-rays may also reveal a raised diaphragm. Computed tomography of the thorax is recommended to exclude mediastinal, pulmonary, or pleural malignancies. Additional abdominal imaging with Doppler sonography is advisable (Benz et al., 2020).

## Recommend Bed Rest During Ascites

Bed rest may encourage diuresis induced by recumbency. Historically, bed rest was advocated under the premise that an upright posture increases plasma renin levels. However, current literature lacks sufficient evidence to routinely recommend bed rest for all clients (Gallo et al., 2020).

**Implement Sodium and Fluid Restriction as Necessary. Ensure Adequate Caloric and Protein Intake**

Sodium restriction helps minimize extravascular fluid retention, while fluid restriction may correct dilutional hyponatremia. Guidelines suggest moderate dietary salt restriction (2 g/day). It is recommended to screen all clients with advanced chronic liver disease for nutritional status and ensure daily energy intake of 35 kcal/kg actual body weight and protein intake of 1.2 to 1.5 g/kg actual body weight to prevent malnutrition (Gallo et al., 2020).

Administer Salt-Free Albumin or Plasma Expanders When Indicated

Albumin increased colloid osmotic pressure in the vascular compartment, drawing fluid back into the vascular space to enhance effective circulating volume and reduce ascites formation. Long-term albumin administration improves effective blood volume by counteracting peripheral arterial vasodilation, preventing renal dysfunction, boosting cardiac contractility, and mitigating systemic inflammation and endothelial dysfunction as an antioxidant (Gallo et al., 2020).

Provide V2 Receptor Antagonists, Inotropes, and Diuretics as Advised

Refer to Pharmacologic Management

## Prepare for Large-Volume Paracentesis as Indicated

Clients with extensive ascites may require large-volume paracentesis to alleviate symptoms such as abdominal discomfort, anorexia, or dyspnea. This procedure can also reduce the risk of umbilical hernia rupture. Large-volume paracentesis is generally considered safe for clients with peripheral edema and those not currently receiving diuretic therapy (Wolf & Anand, 2020).

## Assist in Peritoneovenous Shunt Insertion

Devices like LeVeen and Denver shunts facilitate the return of ascitic fluid and proteins to the intravascular space. Subcutaneously inserted plastic tubing under local anesthesia connects the peritoneal cavity to the internal jugular or subclavian vein via a pumping chamber. These devices effectively alleviate ascites and reverse protein loss in some clients (Wolf & Anand, 2020).

Prepare the Client for Transjugular Intrahepatic Portosystemic Shunt (TIPS) Insertion as Indicated

TIPS is an effective intervention for managing extensive ascites in select clients. TIPS implantation should ideally lower aldosterone, plasma renin, and sinusoidal pressure, which improves sodium excretion through the urine. Multiple studies have demonstrated the superiority of TIPS over large-volume paracentesis in controlling ascites (Wolf & Anand, 2020).

Educate the Client on Medications to Avoid or Use Cautiously

Certain medications pose risks in clients with ascites, such as NSAIDs, which increase sodium retention, hyponatremia, and risk of renal failure. Caution is also advised with metamizole due to its association with persistent acute kidney injury. Drugs like angiotensin-converting enzyme inhibitors, angiotensin II antagonists, and α1-adrenergic receptor blockers should generally be avoided in these clients to mitigate the risk of renal impairment.

## Providing Skin Care and Promoting Skin Integrity

Skin manifestations in systemic disorders provide clues to underlying organ involvement and aid in identifying potential disease-related damage. Skin changes observed in liver cirrhosis are nonspecific and can resemble those seen in non-hepatic disorders. Early identification of cutaneous signs plays a crucial role in preventing or delaying complications and advancing disease stages, thereby reducing morbidity and mortality (Bhandari & Mahajan, 2022).

### Conduct Routine and Detailed Inspection of Pressure Points and Skin Surfaces

Edematous tissues are vulnerable to breakdown and pressure ulcers. Severe cirrhosis-related ascites can stretch the skin, increasing susceptibility to tears. Edema, largely unchanged by positional shifts due to reduced plasma oncotic pressure in liver failure and malabsorption, should be assessed for pitting, tenderness, and associated skin alterations (Goyal et al., 2022).

Monitor for Jaundice, Itching, and Scratching

In hepatic failure, impaired bilirubin excretion leads to its accumulation in skin and sclera, causing jaundice. Bilirubin diffuses into subcutaneous tissues, triggering histamine release and itching. Excessive scratching can exacerbate skin breakdown.

## Implement Gentle Massage and Use Emollient Lotions

Careful skin care is crucial due to subcutaneous edema, client immobility, jaundice, and increased infection susceptibility. Emollient lotions can soothe irritated skin, and efforts should be made to minimize client scratching. Avoiding harsh soaps and adhesive tape helps prevent skin trauma.

## Encourage Regular Repositioning and Assist with Range of Motion (ROM) Exercises

Regular repositioning alleviates pressure on edematous tissues and promotes circulation. ROM exercises improve joint mobility and circulation, benefiting debilitated clients who may require supervised physical therapy programs (Wolf & Anand, 2020).

Recommend Elevating Lower Extremities and Using Compression Stockings

Enhance venous return and reduce edema formation in extremities by elevating legs above heart level for 30 minutes three or four times daily. This may be impractical for individuals with work demands. Prescription compression stockings are essential for moderate to severe edema, prolonged standing, or ulcer management. Effective stockings apply maximum pressure at the ankle, gradually decreasing upwards (Sterns, 2023).

Ensure Linens Remain Dry and Wrinkle-Free

Moisture exacerbates pruritus and increases the risk of skin breakdown. Smooth, wrinkle-free linens reduce friction and roughness, minimizing skin irritation. Dry linens absorb environmental moisture without trapping it against the skin, promoting comfort and skin health.

Recommend Shortening Fingernails and Providing Mittens/Gloves

Short nails prevent inadvertent skin injury, particularly during sleep-induced scratching due to pruritus. Long nails increase the risk of skin trauma during vigorous scratching episodes (Patel et al., 2020).

Provide Perineal Care After Urination and Bowel Movements

Prevent skin breakdown from bile salts with regular perineal care, using mild soap and water followed by barrier cream or ointment application. This routine reduces skin irritation, infection risk, and subsequent complications.

Use Alternating Pressure Mattresses and Other Support Surfaces as Indicated

Reduce dermal pressure, enhance circulation, and mitigate tissue ischemia with appropriate support surfaces. Silicone mattresses, featuring a semisolid material with a silicone outer layer and gel inner layer, conform to body contours, evenly distributing pressure. This design minimizes pressure, shear, and friction on bony prominences, preventing skin damage and pressure ulcer formation (Chen et al., 2022).

Administer Medications Including Cholestyramine, Ursodeoxycholic Acid, Rifampicin, and Selective Serotonin Reuptake Inhibitors (SSRIs) as Indicated.
Refer to Pharmacologic Management for specific indications and dosing guidelines.

Apply Topical Antipruritic Agents Such as Ammonium Lactate Skin Cream as Indicated.
Refer to Pharmacologic Management for recommendations on application and efficacy.

Assist in Preparing the Client for Narrowband Ultraviolet B Therapy (nbUVB).
nbUVB therapy is a common dermatological treatment for itch and inflammatory skin disorders. Its antipruritic effects may result from cytokine modulation, Langerhans cell depletion,

chemical alteration of pruritogens, and reduced skin sensitivity to itch-inducing substances (Patel et al., 2020).

## Managing Respiratory Function and Preventing Pulmonary Complications

Respiratory complications can manifest in clients with or without liver decompensation. These conditions must be differentiated from primary lung diseases like COPD, which may coexist with liver disease but are not causally related to cirrhosis. Common pulmonary complications include hepatic hydrothorax, spontaneous pulmonary empyema, hepatopulmonary syndrome, and portopulmonary hypertension (Benz et al., 2020).

- Monitor Respiratory Rate, Depth, and Effort

Monitor for signs such as rapid shallow breathing or dyspnea, which may indicate hypoxia or abdominal fluid accumulation. Hepatopulmonary syndrome (HPS) is characterized by platypnea (dyspnea relieved by lying down) and orthodeoxia (decrease in arterial oxygen tension upon sitting or standing) (Wolf & Anand, 2020).

- Auscultate Breath Sounds

Listen for crackles, wheezes, and rhonchi, which may indicate developing complications such as fluid accumulation or atelectasis. Hepatic hydrothorax can occur independently of ascites due to negative intrathoracic pressure during inspiration, leading to pleural fluid accumulation instead of abdominal fluid (Benz et al., 2020).

- Assess Level of Consciousness

Changes in mental status may indicate hypoxemia and respiratory failure common in hepatic coma. Hepatic encephalopathy, observed in some cirrhosis clients, presents with personality changes, cognitive impairment, and decreased consciousness. Clients may exhibit deficits in short-term memory and concentration (Wolf & Anand, 2020).

- Monitor Temperature and Respiratory Symptoms

Watch for signs of infection such as chills, increased coughing, and changes in sputum color and consistency, which may indicate pneumonia. Spontaneous bacterial empyema, akin to spontaneous bacterial peritonitis, is a specific complication of hepatic hydrothorax, characterized by fever and symptoms of decompensated liver cirrhosis (Benz et al., 2020).

Optimizing Respiratory Management and Preventing Pulmonary Complications

- Maintain Elevated Head of Bed Position

Keep the head of the bed elevated to alleviate pressure on the diaphragm and reduce the risk of aspiration of secretions. During episodes of dyspnea or orthopnea, assist the client into a semi-Fowler or high-Fowler position. These positions facilitate improved gas exchange, which can be compromised by ascitic fluid exerting pressure on the diaphragm.

- Encourage Regular Repositioning and Breathing Exercises

Promote frequent changes in position and encourage deep-breathing and coughing exercises. These activities aid in lung expansion and help mobilize secretions. Deep breathing expands alveoli and assists in clearing secretions from the airways. Repositioning helps redistribute fluids and mucus in the lungs, reducing the risk of infection and other respiratory complications.

- Provide Oxygen Therapy as Needed

Administer supplemental oxygen to manage or prevent hypoxia. Inadequate oxygenation may necessitate mechanical ventilation. Clients with mild to moderate hepatopulmonary syndrome (HPS) should undergo regular arterial blood gas (ABG) evaluations every 3 to 6 months. Oxygen supplementation is recommended for clients with oxygen saturation below 89% or partial pressure of oxygen less than 55 mm Hg during rest, exercise, and sleep (Surani, 2021).

- Instruct and Assist with Incentive Spirometry or Pulmonary Function Tests

Encourage the use of incentive spirometry to reduce the incidence of atelectasis and facilitate secretion mobilization. Pulmonary function tests should be conducted to assess intrinsic pulmonary disorders. These tests may reveal reduced diffusion capacity for carbon monoxide, indicating impaired gas exchange (Bansal et al., 2022).

Prepare for/Aid with Acute Care Procedures

- Paracentesis

This procedure is occasionally performed to alleviate abdominal pressure caused by ascites when other measures fail to relieve respiratory distress. Large-volume paracentesis is considered safe for clients with peripheral edema and those not currently undergoing diuretic therapy. Studies have demonstrated that 5 to 15 liters of ascitic fluid can be safely removed in one session without significant impact on renal function (Wolf & Anand, 2020).

- Peritoneovenous Shunt

This surgical procedure involves implanting a catheter to redirect accumulated abdominal fluid into the systemic circulation via the vena cava, providing long-term relief from ascites and improving respiratory function. It should be considered a last resort for clients with refractory ascites who are not suitable candidates for TIPS or liver transplantation. Evidence suggests that the safety of repeat large-volume paracentesis may outweigh that of peritoneovenous shunt placement (Wolf & Anand, 2020).

- Transjugular Intrahepatic Portosystemic Shunts (TIPS)

TIPS placement is an effective intervention for managing massive ascites in certain clients. Ideally, it reduces sinusoidal pressure and lowers plasma renin and aldosterone levels, leading to improved urinary sodium excretion. However, TIPS creation may exacerbate pre-existing hepatic encephalopathy and worsen liver function in clients with severe underlying liver disease (Wolf & Anand, 2020).

- Liver Transplantation

For clients with massive ascites, the one-year survival rate is less than 50%. Liver transplantation should be considered as a potential option to rescue the client before irreversible liver failure or hepatorenal syndrome develops (Wolf & Anand, 2020).

- Educate Clients on the Potential Benefits of Garlic in the Diet

Garlic contains allicin, known for its potent vasodilatory and anti-angiogenic properties. Small studies, including randomized controlled trials, suggest that garlic may improve gas exchange. Larger trials are needed to confirm and quantify these benefits (Surani, 2021).

## Enhancing Safety and Preventing Injury

The fibrotic changes that obstruct blood flow through the liver lead to the development of collateral blood vessels within the gastrointestinal (GI) system. This causes blood to bypass the portal vessels and flow into lower-pressure vessels. Consequently, clients with cirrhosis often exhibit prominent distended abdominal vessels visible during abdominal inspection, as well as distended blood vessels throughout the GI tract. Common sites for these vessels include the esophagus, stomach, and lower rectum, where they can form varices or hemorrhoids depending on their location.

Monitor for Signs and Symptoms of GI Bleeding:

Carefully assess all secretions for evidence of frank or occult blood. Monitor the color and consistency of stools, nasogastric drainage, or vomitus. GI bleeding typically arises from the esophagus and rectum due to their mucosal fragility and alterations in hemostasis associated with cirrhosis. The high pressure and volume of blood imposed by cirrhosis on these vessels can cause them to rupture and bleed, necessitating vigilant monitoring for both occult and frank bleeding.

Observe for Petechiae, Ecchymosis, and Bleeding:

Watch for signs of subacute disseminated intravascular coagulation (DIC), which may develop secondary to alterations in clotting factors. Petechiae, ecchymosis, melena, and hematemesis are indicative of bleeding. Significant bleeding may manifest with altered vital signs such as increased heart rate, decreased blood pressure, irritability, air hunger, pallor, and weakness, all of which require prompt intervention.

Monitor Pulse, Blood Pressure, and Central Venous Pressure (if available):

Increased pulse rate coupled with decreased blood pressure and central venous pressure may suggest a loss of circulating blood volume, necessitating further assessment. A study reported that 43% of participants exhibited signs of vital instability upon admission, including hypotension and tachycardia, attributed to portal hypertension causing varices or mucosal changes leading to lower GI bleeding (Khalifa & Rockey, 2020).

Observe Changes in Mentation and Level of Consciousness (LOC):

Changes in mentation or LOC may indicate reduced cerebral perfusion secondary to hypovolemia and hypoxemia. Variceal bleeding can result in hypovolemia and hypotension, impairing oxygen delivery to the brain and potentially causing confusion, disorientation, and altered mental status.

Monitor Hemoglobin, Hematocrit, and Clotting Factors:

Regularly assess hemoglobin and hematocrit levels as well as clotting factors to detect anemia, active bleeding, or impending complications. Due to hypersplenism linked to portal hypertension, poor coagulation, disseminated intravascular coagulation, and hemosiderosis from a variety of reasons, patients with cirrhosis may develop pancytopenia (Farci, 2022).

Avoid Rectal Temperature; Handle GI Tube Insertions with Care

Rectal and esophageal vessels are particularly susceptible to rupture. Avoid invasive procedures such as injections, as clotting alterations in cirrhosis can lead to prolonged bleeding. Thrombocytopenia, caused by increased splenic consumption and decreased platelet production in cirrhosis, significantly heightens the risk of bleeding, especially with platelet counts below 50,000 and in the presence of varices (Flores et al., 2017).

Promote Use of Gentle Oral Care Practices

Encourage the use of a soft toothbrush and electric razor to minimize mucosal trauma. Advise against activities that increase intra-abdominothoracic pressure, such as straining during stool passage, vigorous nose blowing, or heavy lifting, as these can precipitate bleeding episodes in the context of clotting factor disturbances. Hepatic dysfunction disrupts the synthesis of coagulation factors, anticoagulants, fibrinolysis proteins, and platelet regulators, exacerbating the risk of bleeding (Flores et al., 2017).

Use Small Gauge Needles and Apply Prolonged Pressure

Opt for small gauge needles for injections to reduce tissue trauma and potential bleeding. After needle withdrawal, apply pressure to injection sites for an extended period to minimize bleeding and hematoma formation. If bleeding or bruising occurs, consider alternative injection sites to mitigate further complications. Clients with cirrhosis require careful management to prevent exacerbating their underlying clotting dysfunction (Flores et al., 2017).

Caution Against Aspirin Use

Advise against the use of aspirin-containing products due to their potential to prolong coagulation and increase the risk of hemorrhage, particularly in individuals prone to GI bleeding. Despite its efficacy in preventing vascular events, aspirin poses a sustained risk of significant bleeding, prompting caution in guidelines for use among high-risk populations (Mahady et al., 2020).

Administer Medications as Indicated

Administer vitamins, stool softeners, vasoconstrictors, vasodilators, antifibrinolytics, and thrombopoietin agonists based on clinical indications. Refer to the Pharmacologic Management section for specific recommendations.

Perform Gastric Lavage Appropriately

Perform gastric lavage using room temperature saline solution or water in cases of acute bleeding to reduce ammonia production and mitigate the risk of hepatic encephalopathy. Evidence suggests that nasogastric tube (NGT) lavage may expedite endoscopy in bleeding episodes, potentially improving clinical outcomes (Saltzman, 2023).

Assist with Placement and Management of GI Tube

Assist with the insertion and ongoing care of a gastrointestinal (GI) tube. This procedure is utilized temporarily to manage bleeding from esophageal varices when other methods such as lavage are ineffective and hemodynamic stability cannot be achieved. Nasogastric tube (NGT) lavage helps clear particulate matter, fresh blood, and clots from the stomach, facilitating subsequent endoscopic evaluation. It is particularly beneficial when the presence of ongoing bleeding is uncertain and early endoscopy may be advantageous.

Prepare for Surgical Interventions

Prepare for potential surgical procedures such as direct ligation (banding) of varices, esophagogastric resection, or splenorenal-portocaval anastomosis. These interventions may be necessary to control active bleeding or reduce portal and collateral vessel pressures, thereby lowering the risk of recurrent bleeding. Consultations with surgical and interventional radiology teams before endoscopy should be considered based on the likelihood of persistent or recurrent bleeding, or potential risks associated with endoscopic therapies (Sterns, 2023).

## Educate on Dietary Modifications

Educate the client to avoid consuming foods that may irritate or mechanically damage the esophagus, such as rough or spicy foods, hot liquids, and alcohol. A soft diet, comprising easily chewable and swallowable foods, is recommended to minimize esophageal irritation and reduce the risk of bleeding from varices. Specific foods to avoid include taco shells, tortilla chips, hard vegetables like carrot sticks, and large pieces of raw fruit. Encouraging smaller, more frequent meals throughout the day can also help mitigate irritation (Kent, 2017).

## Promote Vitamin K-Rich Foods

Encourage the consumption of foods rich in vitamin K, such as spinach, cabbage, cauliflower, and liver. These foods can help optimize prothrombin time and ensure adequate clotting factor levels, thereby reducing the risk of bleeding episodes. Vitamin K plays a crucial role in blood clotting and can counteract the effects of certain medications like warfarin, helping maintain a balanced clotting function in clients requiring anticoagulant therapy (Kent, 2017).

Administer Blood Products as Prescribed

Administer blood and blood products as prescribed to manage severe anemia and improve hemostasis in cases of bleeding complications associated with cirrhosis.

Transfusion of red blood cells can raise hematocrit levels by more than 25%, enhancing platelet function and clotting ability. Platelet transfusions from pooled donors or apheresis can also significantly increase platelet counts, while off-label use of prothrombin complex concentrates has been noted for correcting vitamin K-dependent clotting factor deficiencies in cirrhotic patients (O'Leary et al., 2019).

## Managing Hepatic Encephalopathy

Hepatic encephalopathy is a syndrome observed in some individuals with cirrhosis, characterized by changes in personality, cognitive impairment, and decreased level of consciousness. The diversion of portal blood into the systemic circulation is believed to be a prerequisite for this condition. Clients may experience altered brain energy metabolism and increased permeability of the blood-brain barrier, potentially facilitating the entry of neurotoxins into the brain (Wolf & Anand, 2020).

### Monitor for Behavioral and Cognitive Changes

Observe signs such as lethargy, confusion, drowsiness, slurred speech, and irritability, as these can indicate fluctuating hepatic coma. Clients with mild to moderate hepatic encephalopathy often exhibit deficits in short-term memory and concentration during mental status assessments (Wolf & Anand, 2020).

Assess Current Medications

Review the client's current medication regimen to identify potential adverse drug reactions and interactions that may exacerbate confusion. For instance, interactions like cimetidine with antacids can potentiate confusion, especially in older adults, those with renal or hepatic impairment, or those receiving high doses of these medications. Additionally, cimetidine can prolong the clearance of benzodiazepines used to manage confusion (Pino & Azer, 2022).

Evaluate Sleep Patterns

Assess the client's sleep and rest schedule to identify any difficulties in falling or staying asleep, which can contribute to cognitive decline and lethargy. Clients with cirrhosis commonly experience sleep disturbances. Medications such as hydroxyzine may improve sleep efficiency and subjective sleep quality, but caution is advised as it may exacerbate encephalopathy in some individuals (Wolf & Anand, 2020).

Monitor for Neurological Signs

Be vigilant for the development or presence of asterixis (flapping tremor), fetor hepaticus (characteristic musty odor of breath), and seizure activity, which may indicate elevated serum ammonia levels and increased risk of encephalopathy progression. Asterixis, although a classic physical finding, can also occur in conditions like uremia, pulmonary insufficiency, and barbiturate toxicity. Clients with portosystemic shunting may exhibit extrapyramidal symptoms such as tremor, bradykinesia, cog-wheel rigidity, and shuffling gait (Wolf & Anand, 2020).

## Managing Hepatic Encephalopathy

Hepatic encephalopathy, observed in some cirrhosis clients, manifests with personality changes, cognitive impairment, and decreased consciousness levels. The diversion of portal blood into the systemic circulation is thought to be a contributing factor. Clients may experience altered brain energy metabolism and increased permeability of the blood-brain barrier, facilitating the passage of neurotoxins into the brain (Wolf & Anand, 2020).

### Consultation with Family Caregivers and Baseline Assessments

Engage family caregivers to assess the client's usual behavior and mental state. Perform baseline evaluations of personality traits, level of consciousness (LOC), and orientation. This establishes a starting point for monitoring any changes in behavior or personality that could progress to hepatic coma if untreated.

Monitoring for Temperature Changes and Signs of Infection

Vigilantly monitor for temperature elevations and signs indicative of infection. Infections can precipitate hepatic encephalopathy by promoting tissue breakdown and nitrogen release, potentially leading to impaired renal function and increased blood ammonia levels. The role of inflammation in conjunction with ammonia suggests diverse anti-inflammatory therapies as potential treatment options for hepatic encephalopathy in cirrhosis clients (Wolf & Anand, 2020).

## Employing Diagnostic Strategies for Hepatic Encephalopathy

Implement testing strategies to detect minimal and covert hepatic encephalopathy, crucial for assessing quality of life and socio-economic implications, and providing guidance to clients and caregivers. The Portosystemic Encephalopathy (PSE) Syndrome Test includes five paper-pencil assessments evaluating cognitive function, psychomotor processing speed, and visual-motor coordination. The Continuous Reaction Times test (CRT) assesses motor reaction time to auditory stimuli, distinguishing between organic and metabolic brain impairments, independent of age or gender, without learning or fatigue effects (Ferenci, 2017).

## Monitoring Writing and Cognitive Function

Regularly have the client write their name for comparison over time. Report any decline in writing ability, as it may indicate worsening hepatic encephalopathy. Characteristics like disorientation and asterixis are indicative of grade 2 hepatic encephalopathy (Wolf & Anand, 2020).

## Promoting Reality Orientation and Creating a Calm Environment

Reorient the client as needed to time, place, and person to reduce confusion and anxiety. This technique aids clients experiencing confusion or disorientation by reconnecting them with their surroundings and current situation.

## Maintaining a Tranquil Environment and Encouraging Rest

Create a serene environment and interact in a calm manner to reduce sensory overload and promote relaxation, potentially enhancing coping mechanisms. Adequate rest reduces the strain on the liver and increases blood supply. As nutritional status improves and strength increases, gradually encourage the client to engage in light activities and exercises, balanced with periods of rest (Wolf & Anand, 2020).

## Ensuring Continuity of Care

If feasible, maintain continuity of care by assigning the same nurse over an extended period. This familiarity provides reassurance, reduces anxiety, and facilitates accurate documentation of subtle changes. Clients who are familiar with their environment and caregivers often feel more secure and less vulnerable, promoting a sense of safety and comfort (Wolf & Anand, 2020).

## Minimizing Provocative Stimuli and Avoiding Confrontation

Minimize provocative stimuli and avoid situations that could lead to confrontation, as these may trigger agitated or violent responses and compromise client safety. Clients with minimal hepatic encephalopathy may retain normal abilities in memory, language, construction, and motor skills, but may experience impairments in complex attention and reaction times (Wolf & Anand, 2020).

## Open Discussion on Current Situation and Future Expectations

Engage in open discussions with the client and their family caregivers about their current situation and what to expect in the future. Providing clear and accurate information can reassure them that cognitive and emotional functions may improve as liver function stabilizes. This communication helps empower clients and caregivers, reducing anxiety and feelings of being overwhelmed by confusion (Wolf & Anand, 2020).

## Promoting Bedrest and Assisting with Self-Care

Encourage bedrest and assist with activities of daily living to minimize metabolic demands on the liver, prevent fatigue, and support healing while reducing the risk of ammonia accumulation. Emphasize the importance of adhering to the comprehensive therapeutic plan, which includes rest, dietary adjustments, and abstaining from alcohol (Wolf & Anand, 2020).

Addressing Safety Needs and Assisting with Ambulation

Identify and address safety needs by assisting with ambulation, ensuring the bed is in a low position, and raising side rails with padding if necessary. This reduces the risk of injury during episodes of confusion, seizures, or agitated behavior. Side rails and padding are essential precautions in case the client becomes restless or agitated due to encephalopathy-related neurosensory changes. Clients undergoing alcohol withdrawal are particularly susceptible to seizures, further necessitating vigilant safety measures (Wolf & Anand, 2020).

Recommendations on Medication Use

Advise against narcotics, sedatives, and anti-anxiety medications, and restrict the use of drugs metabolized by the liver. Some medications are hepatotoxic or may accumulate due to impaired metabolism in cirrhosis, potentially exacerbating encephalopathy or precipitating coma. Avoid central nervous system depressants, especially benzodiazepines. Haloperidol may be considered for sedation in cases of severe agitation and hepatic encephalopathy (Wolf & Anand, 2020).

Dietary Modifications and Hydration

Restrict or eliminate dietary protein intake and provide glucose supplements along with adequate hydration. Ammonia, a byproduct of protein breakdown in the gastrointestinal tract, contributes to mental changes in hepatic encephalopathy. Dietary adjustments aim to minimize constipation, bacterial activity, and ammonia formation. Glucose serves as an energy source, reducing the need for protein catabolism. While protein restriction may be necessary during acute symptom exacerbations, it is generally not warranted in clients with persistent hepatic encephalopathy (Wolf & Anand, 2020).

Promotion of Vegetable Proteins

Encourage consumption of vegetable proteins over animal proteins. Diets rich in vegetable proteins are better tolerated, likely due to higher dietary fiber content and lower levels of aromatic amino acids, which can inhibit dopaminergic neurotransmission and exacerbate hepatic encephalopathy (Wolf & Anand, 2020).

Administration of Therapeutic Agents

Administer cathartics, antibiotics, zinc supplements, and L-ornithine L-aspartate (LOLA) as prescribed. Refer to Pharmacologic Management for specific indications and dosages.

## Promoting Positive Self-Body Image

Living with cirrhosis significantly impacts an individual's quality of life. Health-related quality of life (HRQOL) encompasses perceptions of physical, cognitive, emotional, and social functioning. Research underscores that both physical symptoms and psychological factors profoundly affect HRQOL in individuals with cirrhosis, posing substantial challenges. Disease severity correlates with diminished HRQOL; for instance, ascites can cause discomfort, breathlessness, heightened stress, anxiety related to body image, reduced mobility, and increased fall risks (Polis & Fernandez, 2015).

Facilitating Open Communication and Understanding

Encourage clients to express fears and concerns openly. Clarify how disease progression and symptoms interrelate, particularly regarding changes in body image, which may evoke guilt, especially in cases linked to alcohol or substance use. Managing ascites involves frequent medical procedures, increased medication regimens, and dietary adjustments, all impacting HRQOL (Polis & Fernandez, 2015).

Assessing Changes and Impact

Evaluate changes in appearance and their significance for both the client and their family. This assessment aids in understanding the broader impact on sexual function, role fulfillment, and family dynamics. Clients with cirrhosis commonly experience anxiety, reduced social interactions, delayed treatment, regret, awareness needs, impaired sexual relationships, and financial strain, as evidenced by research participants (Abdi et al., 2015).

## Exploring Coping Strategies

Explore previous coping mechanisms used by the client and family. Encourage the utilization of effective coping strategies previously employed, such as active problem-solving. Studies indicate that sociodemographic factors like gender, family status, or employment status do not significantly influence emotional responses or coping styles among individuals with cirrhosis (Kraus et al., 2000).

## Providing Supportive Care

Support and encourage clients with a compassionate approach. Research highlights instances where individuals with cirrhosis faced discrimination and stigma from healthcare providers, particularly those with a history of alcohol misuse or chronic hepatitis (Brown et al., 2022). Caregivers should strive to provide non-judgmental care, ensuring clients feel valued and respected throughout their care journey.

Supporting Family and Caregivers

Encourage family members and caregivers to openly express their emotions, visit frequently, and actively participate in the client's care. Caregivers often experience guilt and fear about the client's condition, including concerns about mortality. They benefit greatly from empathetic support and unrestricted access to the client, which fosters trust among staff, clients, and caregivers. According to research, support persons play a crucial role in providing practical assistance and encouraging clients to seek necessary medical care (Brown et al., 2022).

Assisting with Changes in Appearance

Assist the client and family caregivers in coping with changes in the client's appearance, such as jaundice, ascites, or bruising. Recommending clothing that minimizes the focus on altered physical features can boost self-esteem and empower the client to maintain a sense of normalcy while exploring adaptive strategies.

Referring to Support Services

Refer clients and caregivers to various support services, counselors, psychiatric resources, social workers, clergy, and alcohol treatment programs as needed. The complex challenges and emotional vulnerabilities associated with cirrhosis often necessitate additional professional support. Access to patient transport services tailored for chronic illness management is crucial for ensuring ongoing healthcare access. Specialist liver nurses play a pivotal role in supporting clients with cirrhosis in self-management and care coordination (Brown et al., 2022).

Setting Short-Term Goals

Assist clients in identifying short-term goals and incorporate them into care planning. Achieving these goals reinforces positive behaviors, enhances self-esteem, and promotes a sense of accomplishment. Insights from studies suggest improving client education through enhanced information dissemination strategies, including informative resources in waiting areas (Brown et al., 2022).

Providing Accurate Information

Provide clients with accurate, tailored information about their condition. Addressing health literacy challenges through visual aids and personalized resources empowers clients to understand and manage their disease effectively, fostering a sense of control over their health (Brown et al., 2022).

## Building Rapport through Effective Communication

Establish a strong rapport with clients and their families through clear, therapeutic communication. Effective communication, particularly in chronic disease management, is critical for achieving positive health outcomes. Strategies may include recruiting culturally competent staff, providing appropriate training, and involving a support person who can facilitate communication during clinical interactions. This approach enhances understanding and collaboration between clients and healthcare professionals.

## Assisting with Recognition of Harmful Practices

Support the client in recognizing past behaviors that may have been detrimental to their health, such as alcohol and drug misuse. Acknowledging the adverse effects of these behaviors is crucial for promoting a path towards a healthier lifestyle. According to findings from a study, individuals with a history of alcohol misuse often acknowledged alcohol as a significant risk factor for cirrhosis, and for some, the diagnosis brought a sense of relief or validation of their concerns. Participants also shared stories of personal resilience that aided them in overcoming alcohol dependency (Brown et al., 2022).

## Initiating Patient Education and Health Teachings

Cirrhosis profoundly impacts patients' lives and extends its effects to their families and society at large. When a family member falls ill, it affects all members. Therefore, educating these patients becomes imperative to manage their condition effectively, mitigate complications, and maintain their quality of life (Abdi et al., 2015). Managing cirrhosis optimally is intricate, and empowering patients with the necessary knowledge enhances the efficacy of chronic disease management (Brown et al., 2022).

### Review of Disease Process, Prognosis, and Future Expectations

This session provides foundational knowledge enabling clients to make informed decisions. **Health literacy** refers to individuals' capacity to acquire, process, and comprehend essential health-related information necessary for making appropriate health decisions (Brown et al., 2022).

Identification of Environmental Risks, such as Hepatitis Exposure

Exposure to hepatitis can precipitate disease recurrence. While alcoholic liver disease was once predominant in the United States, hepatitis C has now emerged as the leading cause of chronic hepatitis and cirrhosis (Wolf & Anand, 2020).

Assessment of Client Awareness and Knowledge Regarding Disease and Treatment

The level of awareness and knowledge clients possess about their disease can significantly impact their treatment experience. Research indicates that patients with hepatocellular carcinoma actively seek information about their condition (Abdi et al., 2015).

Assessment of Client Anxiety Levels

From a healthcare provider's perspective, initial anxiety at the time of diagnosis presents an opportunity to initiate behavioral change and motivate clients. Studies suggest that high levels of anxiety can enhance clients' readiness to absorb information and modify lifestyle habits, highlighting the importance of early educational interventions (Abdi et al., 2015).

Referral to Dietitian or Nutritionist

Clients with cirrhosis require close monitoring and comprehensive nutritional guidance. During hospitalization, nurses and healthcare providers prepare cirrhosis patients for discharge, emphasizing dietary education. Avoiding alcohol consumption is paramount, and clients may benefit from referrals to Alcoholics Anonymous, psychiatric counseling, or spiritual support (Abdi et al., 2015).

Emphasize the Importance of Alcohol Avoidance and Provide Information on Alcohol Rehabilitation Services

Alcohol consumption stands as the primary cause of cirrhosis development. In a study, participants shared experiences of alcohol cessation and counseling, with some highlighting personal resilience in abstaining from alcohol. However, counseling was perceived as daunting by some, particularly discussing alcohol misuse in group settings. Others expressed interest but noted limited access to counseling services in their locality (Brown et al., 2022).

Educate Clients on the Effects of Medications in Cirrhosis and the Importance of Medical Supervision

Certain medications, notably narcotics, sedatives, and hypnotics, can be hepatotoxic. Moreover, impaired liver function diminishes drug metabolism capability, potentially leading to cumulative effects or increased bleeding risks. Introducing any new therapy mandates frequent liver function monitoring to prevent drug-induced liver complications, which could exacerbate existing liver disease (Wolf & Anand, 2020).

Review Maintenance Procedures for Peritoneovenous Shunt Function

For clients with a Denver shunt, regular chamber pumping is necessary to maintain device patency. Conversely, those with a LeVeen shunt may use an abdominal binder or perform a Valsalva maneuver to support shunt functionality. Both shunts facilitate the return of ascites fluid and proteins into the bloodstream via subcutaneously inserted plastic tubing connected to the internal jugular or subclavian vein, enhancing intravascular fluid balance (Wolf & Anand, 2020).

Assist the Client in Identifying Support Persons

Given the prolonged recovery period, potential for relapse, and gradual convalescence, support systems are crucial for sustaining behavioral changes. Clients highlighted the significant role of support persons in providing practical assistance and encouraging adherence to medical care (Brown et al., 2022).

Emphasize the Importance of Optimal Nutrition

Maintaining a proper diet, avoiding high-protein and salty foods, as well as onions and strong cheeses, supports symptom remission and helps prevent ammonia buildup and further liver damage. Providing written dietary guidelines aids clients in managing their diet effectively at home. Clients without ascites, edema, or impending hepatic coma should aim for a nutritious, high-protein diet supplemented with B complex, vitamins A, C, and K, while also limiting sodium intake to prevent ascites formation.

Stress the Necessity of Follow-up Care and Treatment Adherence

Given the chronicity of the disease and potential for life-threatening complications, regular follow-up is essential to assess treatment effectiveness, including shunt patency where applicable. Client cooperation with the therapeutic plan—comprising rest, lifestyle adjustments, proper nutrition, and alcohol cessation—is crucial for successful management.

## Discuss Sodium and Salt Substitute Restrictions

Managing sodium intake and avoiding salt substitutes helps minimize ascites and edema. Caution is advised regarding potential electrolyte imbalances from excessive substitute use. Clients should diligently check food and over-the-counter drug labels, as products like antacids and mouthwashes may contain sodium or alcohol. The nutritional benefits of commercial liquid supplements, despite moderate sodium content, often outweigh the risk of slightly increased salt intake (Wolf & Anand, 2020).

Encourage Scheduling Activities with Adequate Rest Periods

Ensuring sufficient rest reduces metabolic demands on the body and enhances energy available for tissue regeneration. Rest also reduces strain on the liver and improves its blood supply, crucial for clients vulnerable to complications of immobility such as respiratory, circulatory, and vascular disturbances. These measures help prevent issues like atelectasis, pneumonia, venous thromboembolism, and pressure ulcers.

Promote Enjoyable Diversional Activities

Engaging in enjoyable activities prevents boredom and reduces anxiety and depression, which can impact various aspects of cirrhosis care, including medication adherence, self-care, engagement with healthcare services, and risk behaviors such as alcohol misuse. Addressing psychological needs through diversional activities and psychosocial counseling can provide essential mental health support (Brown et al., 2022).

Recommend Avoidance of Individuals with Infections, Particularly Upper Respiratory Infections

Reduced resistance and altered immune response increase susceptibility to infections, exacerbated by factors like anemia and poor nutritional status. Clients with cirrhosis face a heightened risk of bacterial infections and sepsis during hospitalization, underscoring the importance of infection prevention (Tonon et al., 2021).

Educate on Signs and Symptoms Requiring Prompt Healthcare Provider Notification

Clients and caregivers should promptly report symptoms such as increased abdominal girth, rapid weight changes, peripheral edema, dyspnea, fever, and signs of bleeding or jaundice. Early reporting mitigates hepatic damage and allows timely intervention to prevent life-threatening complications, including bleeding and hemorrhage due to impaired liver function.

Instruct Caregivers to Monitor and Report Changes in Mental Status

Changes such as confusion, disorientation, tremors, or personality changes should be reported promptly. Careful monitoring helps detect early signs of mental status deterioration, crucial for timely intervention and ongoing neurological assessment to manage hepatic encephalopathy effectively.

Prepare Clients and Caregivers for Transitional Care

Transitioning from hospital to home care requires preparation and ongoing support. Referral to transitional or home care services facilitates adjustment to new routines, including dietary and lifestyle changes. Nurses play a vital role in reinforcing previous education, addressing emerging questions, and supporting clients and families during this critical phase of care.

Supporting Recovery and Encouraging Clients and Families

Navigating recovery poses challenges, characterized by slow progress, setbacks, and periods of perceived stagnation. Many individuals find it challenging to resist using alcohol for comfort or escape. Nurses play a pivotal role in providing unwavering support and encouragement to clients, alongside offering positive reinforcement during moments of success.

## Administering Medications and Providing Pharmacologic Support

Medications prescribed for patients with liver cirrhosis aim to manage the underlying liver disease, prevent complications, and alleviate symptoms. Treatment may include diuretics such as spironolactone or furosemide to address ascites and edema, lactulose or rifaximin for hepatic encephalopathy, beta-blockers like propranolol or nadolol to reduce variceal bleeding risk, and ursodeoxycholic acid to enhance bile flow and protect liver cells.

## Oral Branched Chain Amino Acids (BCAA) Preparations

To address hypoalbuminemia and amino acid imbalances, oral BCAA preparations are beneficial. These preparations, including granules and enteral nutrients, should be administered based on the nutritional status and presence of hepatic encephalopathy. Administering BCAA granules helps maintain or elevate serum albumin levels in patients with decompensated liver cirrhosis, improving prognosis and enhancing quality of life (Yoshiji & Kaji, 2019).

Diuretics: Spironolactone and Furosemide

These medications are cautiously employed to manage edema and ascites by blocking aldosterone's effects and promoting water excretion while preserving potassium. In hospitalized patients with severe ascites, aggressive diuretic therapy can safely induce daily weight loss of 0.5 to 1 kg under close monitoring of renal function. Therapy should be interrupted if electrolyte imbalances, azotemia, or hepatic encephalopathy occur (Wolf & Anand, 2020).

Positive Inotropic Drugs and Arterial Vasodilators

These medications are administered to enhance cardiac output and improve renal blood flow, thereby reducing fluid retention. Non-selective beta-blockers (NSBBs) decrease portal pressure and are currently utilized for both primary and secondary prevention of variceal hemorrhage. Studies indicate that NSBBs may also offer protective benefits in patients with decompensated cirrhosis by reducing intestinal permeability and inflammation at advanced stages (Gallo et al., 2020).

V2 Receptor Antagonists

Vasopressin receptor antagonists belong to a class of agents designed to increase free-water excretion, enhance diuresis, and potentially reduce the need for paracentesis. However, no V2 receptor antagonist has received approval from the US Food and Drug Administration (FDA) for this specific indication. Tolvaptan, an oral V2 receptor antagonist, gained FDA approval in 2009 solely for managing hyponatremia (Wolf & Anand, 2020).

Cholestyramine

Cholestyramine, an anion exchange resin, remains the first-line treatment recommended in guidelines for pruritus associated with liver diseases. It is typically administered as a 4-gram sachet, taken one hour before and after breakfast. Patients should be advised to allow at least a 4-hour interval between taking cholestyramine and any other medications to prevent potential interference with intestinal absorption (Düll & Kremer, 2019).

Ursodeoxycholic Acid

Ursodeoxycholic acid (UDCA) is a bile acid used as foundational therapy in various cholestatic conditions, significantly improving overall survival rates. Research shows that UDCA, at doses ranging from 13 to 15 mg/kg/day, notably reduces pruritus severity, particularly in women. A recent meta-analysis of 11 randomized controlled trials highlighted that 73% of women experienced improved pruritus with UDCA therapy (Düll & Kremer, 2019).

### Rifampicin

As a second-line treatment for pruritus resulting from liver disease, rifampicin is advised. Besides its antibiotic properties, rifampicin can modify the intestinal and skin microbiome. It is well-tolerated over long durations and has demonstrated strong anti-itch effects in hepatic pruritus. Regular laboratory monitoring is essential during therapy, particularly at 6 and 12 weeks, to monitor for potential hepatotoxicity, a serious side effect (Düll & Kremer, 2019).

### Selective Serotonin Reuptake Inhibitors (SSRIs)

SSRIs can be considered a fifth-line treatment option for pruritus. In a single placebo-controlled, cross-over trial, sertraline demonstrated a moderate reduction in itching. Recommended dosages for sertraline range from 75 to 100 mg/day (Düll & Kremer, 2019).

Topical Antipruritic Agents

For mild itching associated with liver cirrhosis, topical ammonium lactate skin cream can be effective. A 12% ammonium lactate lotion is recommended for temporary relief from pruritus.

Supplemental Vitamins

Supplementing with vitamins K, D, and C can be beneficial for patients with liver issues. Vitamin

K supports prothrombin synthesis and coagulation, while vitamin C helps reduce gastrointestinal irritation and bleeding risks. Care should be taken with vitamin A and iron supplements due to their potential hepatotoxicity and difficulty in processing high doses, respectively (Daniel, 2022).

Stool Softeners

Stool softeners help prevent straining during bowel movements, thereby reducing the risk of vascular rupture and hemorrhage. Lactulose is also beneficial for patients with hepatic encephalopathy as it aids in moving ammonia from tissues into the gut (Wolf & Anand, 2020).

Vasodilators

Vasodilators are advantageous in treating variceal bleeding in emergency settings. They help lower portal pressure and provide a clearer view of varices for endoscopists by reducing active bleeding (Carale & Anand, 2017).

Antifibrinolytics

Aminocaproic acid and tranexamic acid are used to reduce hyperfibrinolysis over short durations, administered orally or intravenously. Aminocaproic acid is given at 3 g orally four times daily until bleeding is controlled, while tranexamic acid is recommended at 1 g IV every 6 hours. These agents are typically employed as rescue measures rather than for prophylaxis (O'Leary et al., 2019).

I

Vasoconstrictors

Somatostatin and octreotide are vasoconstrictors used to manage acute bleeding in patients with portal hypertension prior to endoscopy. Intravenous infusions of octreotide can lower portal blood pressure and help prevent rebleeding during the initial hospitalization period (Carale & Anand, 2017).

Thrombopoietin Agonists

Avatrombopag and lusutrombopag are oral thrombopoietin agonists that have completed phase 3 trials and received US FDA approval for use in patients with liver disease. These agents can be administered short-term in chronic liver disease to increase platelet counts before invasive procedures (O'Leary et al., 2019).

## Cathartics

Lactulose and lactitol, non-absorbable disaccharides used since the early 1970s, are broken down by intestinal bacteria into lactic acid and other organic acids. These compounds inhibit intestinal ammonia production and reduce colonic bacterial load (Wolf & Anand, 2020).

## Antibiotics

Neomycin, along with other antibiotics like metronidazole, oral vancomycin, paromomycin, and oral quinolones, is used to decrease the concentration of ammonia-producing bacteria in the colon. Neomycin is typically a second-line treatment after lactulose. Rifaximin, a nonabsorbable derivative of rifampin, is as effective as lactulose or lactitol in alleviating symptoms of hepatic encephalopathy.

L-Ornithine L-Aspartate (LOLA)

LOLA, available in Europe but not the United States, is a stable salt of two amino acids. L-ornithine stimulates the urea cycle, leading to the reduction of ammonia levels. European trials have demonstrated LOLA's effectiveness in treating hepatic encephalopathy (Wolf & Anand, 2020).

Zinc

Zinc supplementation can improve hyperammonemia by enhancing the activity of ornithine transcarbamylase, an enzyme involved in the urea cycle. This increase in ureagenesis results in the elimination of ammonia ions. Clinical trials have used zinc sulfate and zinc acetate at a dose of 600 mg orally per day (Wolf & Anand, 2020).

## Monitoring Diagnostic and Laboratory Results

For patients with liver cirrhosis, laboratory tests such as liver function tests (ALT, AST, bilirubin, albumin, and INR) are essential to evaluate liver function and the extent of liver damage. Additional tests like complete blood count, renal function tests, viral hepatitis serology, and imaging studies (ultrasound or CT scan) are conducted to further assess the liver and identify underlying causes or complications associated with cirrhosis.

Serum Glucose, Prealbumin, Albumin, Total Protein, Prothrombin Time (PT), and Ammonia

Glucose levels may be reduced due to impaired gluconeogenesis, depleted glycogen stores, or inadequate intake. Protein levels might be low due to impaired metabolism, decreased hepatic synthesis, or loss into the peritoneal cavity (ascites). Elevated ammonia levels may necessitate protein intake restrictions to prevent serious complications. PT is elevated due to coagulation factor defects, while bilirubin and albumin levels are low, reflecting the liver's declining functional capacity. Therefore, serum albumin and PT are reliable indicators of hepatic synthetic function (Farci, 2022).

ABGs, Pulse Oximetry, Vital Capacity Measurements, and Chest X-rays

These tests detect changes in respiratory status, indicating potential pulmonary complications. Pulse oximetry, with a cutoff of 96% saturation at room air, serves as an initial screening test. An SpO2 <96% is highly sensitive and specific for detecting hepatopulmonary syndrome (HPS) in patients with a PaO2 <70 mm Hg. Patients with HPS typically show normal spirometry and lung volume measurements. In ABG analysis, HPS is classified by the degree of hypoxemia: mild (PaO2 >80 mm Hg), moderate (PaO2 60 to 79 mm Hg), severe (PaO2 50 to 59 mm Hg), and very severe (PaO2 <50 mm Hg) (Benz et al., 2020).

## Monitoring Diagnostic and Laboratory Results

For patients with liver cirrhosis, laboratory tests are crucial to assess liver function and determine the severity of liver damage. These tests include liver function tests (ALT, AST, bilirubin, albumin, and INR). Additional evaluations, such as complete blood count, renal function tests, viral hepatitis serology, and imaging studies (ultrasound or CT scan), may be performed to further investigate the liver and identify any underlying causes or complications related to cirrhosis.

Serum Glucose, Prealbumin, Albumin, Total Protein, Prothrombin Time (PT), and Ammonia

Decreased glucose levels can result from impaired gluconeogenesis, depleted glycogen stores, or inadequate intake. Protein levels may be low due to impaired metabolism, decreased hepatic synthesis, or loss into the peritoneal cavity (ascites). Elevated ammonia levels may necessitate protein intake restrictions to prevent serious complications. PT is elevated due to defects in coagulation factors, while bilirubin and albumin levels are low, reflecting the liver's declining synthetic capacity. Thus, serum albumin and PT are reliable indicators of hepatic synthetic function (Farci, 2022).

ABGs, Pulse Oximetry, Vital Capacity Measurements, and Chest X-rays

These tests are used to detect changes in respiratory status and identify potential pulmonary complications. Pulse oximetry, with a cutoff of 96% saturation at room air, serves as an initial screening tool. An SpO2 <96% is highly sensitive and specific for detecting hepatopulmonary syndrome (HPS) in patients with a PaO2 <70 mm Hg. Patients with HPS typically show normal spirometry and lung volume measurements. In ABG analysis, HPS is classified by the degree of hypoxemia: mild (PaO2 >80 mm Hg), moderate (PaO2 60 to 79 mm Hg), severe (PaO2 50 to 59 mm Hg), and very severe (PaO2 <50 mm Hg) (Benz et al., 2020).

Renal Function Tests

Hepatorenal syndrome is diagnosed when a creatinine clearance rate of less than 40 mL/minute is present or when a serum creatinine level exceeds 1.5 mg/dL, urine volume is less than 500 mL/day, and urine sodium levels are below 10 mEq/L. Urine osmolality is typically higher than plasma osmolality in such cases (Wolf & Anand, 2020).

Contrast-Enhanced Echocardiography

To diagnose pulmonary vascular dilatation, the gold standard is contrast-enhanced echocardiography using agitated saline. This procedure involves agitating normal saline to create microbubbles larger than 10 micrometers in diameter. The agitated saline is then injected into a peripheral vein in the arm while simultaneous transthoracic echocardiography (TTE) is performed. The presence of microbubbles in the left atrium between the 4th and 6th cardiac cycles signifies pulmonary vasodilatation (Bansal et al., 2022).

Dear Reader,

Your experience matters! If you've found "Mastering Liver Cirrhosis: A Comprehensive Guide to Nursing Care Plans and Management" insightful and helpful, please consider sharing your thoughts in a review. Your feedback not only helps other readers discover valuable insights but also guides us in continuously improving our resources to better serve you.

Thank you for being part of our journey in enhancing heart failure care through knowledge and compassion.

Warm regards,

Dr. Roy B. Vicknair